HERBAL REMEDIES FOR IBS

Harmony Through Herbs For Sustainable Relief, Holistic Wellness, Targeted Healing And Reclaiming Gut Health

DR. CARDEN KYRIE

DISCLAIMER

The only goal of this book is informational. Every effort has been taken by the author and publisher to ensure that the information provided is accurate. But the material in this book is given "as is," without any express or implied representation, warranty, or condition as to its accuracy, completeness, or suitability for any particular purpose.

Any loss, damage, or injury resulting from using the information in this book, or from any action or decision made as a result of such use, will not be covered by the author's or publisher's liability. It is recommended that readers seek the assistance of a certified specialist for guidance specific to their situation.

The opinions and viewpoints conveyed in this book belong to the author and may not necessarily represent the official stance or policies of any specified organizations or people. Any likeness to real-life occurrences, places, or people—living or deceased—is wholly coincidental.

No specific product, service, or therapy discussed in this book is endorsed by the author or publisher. Any reference to goods or services is made only for informative reasons and is not intended as a recommendation or endorsement.

Before making any judgments or acting on any information, readers are urged to independently confirm it all. Any unfavorable effects or repercussions arising from the usage of the material included in this book are disclaimed by the author and publisher.

By using this book, you consent to absolving the publisher and author of any and all claims, obligations, or losses resulting from your use of the material in it.

I appreciate your cooperation and understanding.

TABLE OF CONTENTS

CHAPTER ONE

INTRODUCTION TO IBS

CONCERNING IBS, OR INFLAMMATORY BOWEL SYNDROME

The complicated and long-lasting gastrointestinal ailment known as Inflammatory Bowel Syndrome (IBS) has a substantial negative influence on the quality of life of individuals who have it. Since this syndrome is not a discrete disease but rather a collection of symptoms, medical experts may find it difficult to diagnose and treat this syndrome. The similarities in symptoms between IBS and other gastrointestinal disorders, like inflammatory bowel disease (IBD), make diagnosis more difficult.

DEFINITION AND SYNOPSIS

Fundamentally, IBS is characterized by disruptions in the regular operation of the gastrointestinal system, which result in a range of painful and occasionally incapacitating symptoms. These symptoms might include bloating and soreness in the abdomen as well as changes in bowel habits, such as constipation, diarrhea, or both. IBS is a difficult disorder that necessitates a thorough understanding of optimal care because of its wide and unpredictable range of symptoms.

TYPICAL SYMPTOMS

Understanding the many symptoms of IBS is essential to understanding the condition. A defining characteristic of abdominal pain is cramping and discomfort that can vary in severity. Another common symptom that adds to the general pain that people with IBS feel is bloating. Additionally, the illness presents as alterations in bowel habits; some patients have diarrhea, some have constipation, and some alternate between the two. The disorder can be difficult to manage because of the erratic nature of these symptoms, which can make daily life for people who are impacted unpredictable.

REASONS AND INITIATORS

Examining the origins and stimulants of IBS helps to clarify the complex nature of this condition. Although the precise cause of IBS is still unknown, it is generally acknowledged that several factors have a role in both its onset and aggravation. These include modifications to the gut microbiota, increased visceral sensitivity, and abnormalities in the motility of the gastrointestinal tract. Stress and anxiety are examples of psychological elements that are acknowledged as possible causes. The identification of a single causal agent can be made more difficult by the potential for particular dietary components and food sensitivities to function as triggers.

IBS symptoms can have a wide variety of unique triggers. Certain foods can cause symptoms in some people, including dairy, spicy meals, and artificial sweeteners. Stress and other emotional variables can also significantly exacerbate symptoms, emphasizing the complex interaction between the brain and the gut in IBS. Comprehending these triggers is essential to creating efficient management plans customized to each person's unique requirements.

Inflammatory bowel syndrome is a complex gastrointestinal disorder with a wide range of symptoms, including bloating and pain in the abdomen as well as irregular bowel movements. A comprehensive approach to diagnosis and management is required due to the mysterious nature of its triggers and causes. With the growing comprehension of the complex interactions of genetic, environmental, and psychological factors, we can create more individualized and focused interventions for people struggling with IBS.

CHAPTER TWO

THE VALUE OF NATURAL TREATMENTS

A COMPREHENSIVE APPROACH TO IBS

When treating Irritable Bowel Syndrome (IBS), a holistic approach highlights the connection between many facets of health, such as mental, emotional, and physical health. In contrast to traditional treatment, which frequently concentrates on addressing certain symptoms, a holistic approach to IBS seeks to address the underlying causes of the illness. This method recognizes that IBS is a complicated illness impacted by a variety of variables, including lifestyle, diet, stress, and mental well-being.

A holistic approach to treating IBS takes into account the functions of the entire digestive system as well as potential causes. This entails evaluating eating patterns, detecting dietary sensitivity, controlling stress, and fostering a balanced gut flora. The significance of individualized treatment programs that consider the particular requirements and experiences of each IBS patient is frequently emphasized by holistic practitioners.

ADVANTAGES OF NATURAL TREATMENTS

Numerous advantages of using natural treatments for IBS align with the ideas of holistic healing. The reduction of adverse effects that are frequently linked to medicinal interventions is a noteworthy benefit. Numerous natural treatments, including dietary adjustments, lifestyle alterations, and herbal supplements, seek to bring the body back into balance while avoiding negative side effects. Furthermore, these treatments frequently support the body's natural functions, encouraging a kinder and more long-term approach to treating IBS symptoms.

The ability of natural therapies to address several elements of health at once is another advantage. For instance, dietary modifications emphasizing complete, unadulterated meals promote general well-being and digestive health. Herbal therapies can address both the physical and emotional aspects of IBS by relaxing the digestive system and encouraging relaxation. Examples of these remedies include peppermint oil and chamomile tea.

COMBINING MEDICAL CARE WITH NATURAL THERAPIES

The combination of traditional medical treatment for IBS with natural remedies represents a complementary strategy aimed at improving patient results. Although some people may require medical interventions like prescription pharmaceuticals, using natural therapies can improve the treatment plan's overall efficacy.

Working together, medical professionals conventional physicians as well as holistic healers can give patients a thorough and all-encompassing approach to controlling IBS. For example, a gastroenterologist might provide drugs to treat a particular ailment, but a nutritionist or herbalist could advise on dietary adjustments and vitamins to maintain digestive health.

The use of herbal remedies in medical care is significant because it recognizes the value of personalized care. One person's solution might not be appropriate for another, and a customized strategy gives you flexibility in treating the various aspects that contribute to IBS. Patients may benefit from a more all-encompassing and long-lasting strategy for managing their IBS symptoms by combining the benefits of conventional treatment with natural medicines, promoting long-term well-being.

CHAPTER THREE

KNOWLEDGE OF INFLAMMATORY BOWEL DISEASE

IBS TYPES

Manifestations of a common gastrointestinal condition affecting the large intestine include Inflammatory Bowel Syndrome (IBS). It's a long-term illness that can seriously lower someone's quality of life. A noteworthy feature of IBS is that it may be divided into several varieties, each identified by the symptoms that predominate in each type. IBS-C (constipation-predominant), IBS-D (diarrhea-predominant), and IBS-M (mixed) are the three primary forms of IBS.

IBS-C (PREDOMINANTLY CONSTIPATED)

Constipation-predominant IBS, often known as IBS-C, is typified by infrequent bowel motions and trouble passing stool. After a bowel movement, people with this subtype frequently report bloating, abdominal pain, and a feeling of incomplete evacuation. IBS-C sufferers may also have straining during bowel movements in addition to constipation, which adds to the discomfort of the condition overall.

IBS-D, or diarrhea-predominant IBS, on the other hand, is characterized by frequent, loose, or watery feces. People who have IBS-D may have frequent, urgent bowel movements, which makes them more frequent bathroom users. This subtype is frequently linked to cramping and pain in the abdomen. For patients with this type of IBS, the unexpected nature of diarrhea can have a substantial influence on everyday activities and perhaps exacerbate feelings of stress or anxiety.

DIARRHEA-PREDOMINANT IBS-D

Constipation and diarrhea symptoms are combined in IBS-M, or Mixed IBS, a variant of the illness. People who have IBS-M frequently have stomach pain or discomfort and may alternate between episodes of diarrhea and constipation. It can be difficult to control the oscillation between two opposed symptoms, necessitating a multifaceted approach to treatment that takes into account both facets of the illness.

IBS-M (UNDIVIDED)

Although the precise origin of IBS is still unknown, several factors, such as heredity, food, gut motility, and sensitivity to specific stimuli, are probably involved. Healthcare providers can more effectively customize treatment plans to target the unique symptoms that predominate in each patient according to the subtype classification.

A multidisciplinary approach, including dietary adjustments, lifestyle changes, and medication, is frequently used in the management of IBS. For those with symptoms predominating in constipation, dietary fiber, probiotics, and drugs affecting gut motility may be advised; for those with symptoms predominating in diarrhea, anti-diarrheal medications and dietary modifications are typical. For people with mixed IBS, lifestyle adjustments, stress reduction methods, and therapy may be helpful.

Medical practitioners must comprehend the various forms of IBS to create treatment regimens that work and for IBS sufferers to be able to better control their symptoms. It is hoped that new and more tailored medicines will emerge as research into the underlying mechanisms of IBS continues, providing better comfort for those suffering from this difficult ailment.

CHAPTER FOUR

IDENTIFICATION AND ASSESSMENT
TYPICAL DIAGNOSTIC TECHNIQUES

In the medical field, a precise diagnosis is essential to a successful course of treatment. Common diagnostic techniques are essential for identifying the underlying causes of a wide range of medical disorders. Of them, medical imaging—which includes methods like MRIs, CT scans, and X-rays—stands out as a major participant. These non-invasive techniques offer thorough insights into the body's internal components, making it easier to spot anomalies, wounds, or illnesses.

Diagnostic processes also include laboratory testing as a crucial component. Tests such as blood, urine, and genetics provide important details about a patient's health. Biochemical imbalances, genetic predispositions, or the presence of particular markers suggestive of particular diseases can all be revealed by the results. These diagnostic tools enable medical professionals to decide on treatment strategies with knowledge.

RECOGNIZING TRIGGERS

Finding triggers is an essential part of the diagnostic process, particularly in cases when symptoms are influenced by outside variables. Triggers are situations or stimuli that have the power to initiate or worsen a medical condition. When it comes to allergies, for example, identifying particular allergens is crucial. This includes conducting a thorough medical history, testing for allergies, and monitoring symptom trends.

Finding the origins of mental health disorders like anxiety and depression entails examining traumatic events, environmental stresses, and metabolic imbalances. Open communication and trust are fostered between patients and healthcare providers, as this procedure frequently calls for their cooperation.

TRADITIONAL THERAPIES

Conventional therapies serve as the cornerstone of medical intervention and are frequently the initial course of treatment for a variety of medical ailments. These therapies cover a wide range of options, including medication, lifestyle changes, and surgery. Traditional methods have been shown safe and effective through extensive testing and evidence-based practices.

DRUGS

Pharmacotherapy is essential for treating a wide range of illnesses. Drugs can be created to treat infections, control chronic illnesses, or lessen symptoms. In certain situations, reestablishing the body's equilibrium by physiological process modulation is the aim. When prescribing medication, a patient's medical history, current conditions, and possible drug interactions are all carefully taken into account.

CHANGES IN LIFESTYLE

Lifestyle changes are frequently essential parts of an all-encompassing therapeutic program. These adjustments may involve food alterations, workout plans, stress reduction strategies, and sleep schedule adjustments. When it comes to disorders like obesity, diabetes, and cardiovascular disease, where habits and behaviors have a big influence on general health, lifestyle therapies are especially important.

SURGICAL SOLUTIONS

Surgical options may be taken into consideration in circumstances of acute medical emergency or when conservative methods are shown to be insufficient. Surgical interventions can vary in complexity and type, based on the type and severity of the underlying medical issue. These can include minimally invasive treatments. Surgery is frequently used to treat diseases that cannot be effectively treated non-invasively, remove tumors, and fix structural abnormalities.

CHAPTER FIVE

NATURAL METHODS FOR HANDLING IBS

Dietary adjustments are essential for the management of Irritable Bowel Syndrome (IBS), providing a non-invasive means of symptom relief and improving general health. Taking into account the kinds and quantities of fiber in one's diet is one important component. Because fiber promotes regular bowel movements and helps control the symptoms of irritable bowel syndrome, it is crucial for digestive health. It's crucial to find a balance, though, as some people may have worsening symptoms from consuming too much fiber. It's critical to customize fiber intake based on personal needs to achieve optimal digestive function.

The Specific Carbohydrate Diet (SCD) is an additional dietary strategy that is becoming more popular for treating IBS. To relieve gastrointestinal problems, the main goal of this regimen is to restrict specific complex carbs.

Following the SCD aims to lessen intestinal irritation and improve overall digestive health by restricting the consumption of certain carbohydrates that may be difficult to digest. Understanding that different people may have different triggers for their IBS symptoms, SCD can be viewed as a tailored strategy.

Another dietary approach that is becoming more well-acknowledged for its efficacy in treating IBS symptoms is the Low FODMAP Diet. Fermentable Oligosaccharides, Disaccharides, Monosaccharides, and Polyols, or FODMAPs, are a class of carbohydrates that, in sensitive people, may cause symptoms related to the digestive system. Restricting foods high in these fermentable carbohydrates is part of the Low FODMAP Diet, which aims to lessen symptoms including gas, bloating, and stomach pain. It is a sophisticated method that entails meticulous food identification and exclusion, then a methodical reintroduction phase to ascertain each person's threshold levels.

Because triggers can differ greatly across people, implementing dietary adjustments for the management of IBS requires a thorough and personalized approach. A higher fiber diet may help some people feel better, while the Low FODMAP Diet or the Specific Carbohydrate Diet may provide more focused benefits for others. IBS sufferers must collaborate closely with medical specialists and/or qualified dietitians to develop a customized eating plan that takes into account their unique symptoms and dietary requirements.

Dietary modifications combined with natural methods of managing IBS provide a potentially effective way to alleviate symptoms. Gaining knowledge about the benefits of fiber, delving into the subtleties of the Specific Carbohydrate Diet, and embracing the Low FODMAP Diet can enable people to actively manage their digestive health. With individualized and knowledgeable dietary decisions, people with IBS can reduce symptoms and enhance their general quality of life.

CHAPTER SIX

HERBAL TREATMENTS

ALOE VERA

For generations, people have valued the medical benefits of aloe vera, a succulent plant with thick, meaty leaves. Its leaf gel is a multipurpose medicinal that may be used for anything from digestive health to skin care. Aloe vera, which is abundant in vitamins, minerals, and antioxidants, is well known for its capacity to calm and moisturize skin. Because of its anti-inflammatory and antibacterial qualities, it is frequently used to treat sunburns, wounds, and other skin disorders.

Aloe vera is prized for its possible digestive advantages in addition to its cosmetic uses. Compounds having laxative properties can be discovered in the yellowish material called latex, which is located directly beneath the leaf skin. Aloe vera has been traditionally used to treat constipation, but it must be handled carefully when used for digestive issues because too much of it might have negative effects. Furthermore, research is still being done to see whether it can help manage disorders including inflammatory bowel disease and diabetes, but more research is required to draw firm conclusions.

PEPPERMINT OIL

The peppermint plant yields peppermint oil, a popular herbal treatment with a wide range of health advantages. Its main active ingredient, menthol, gives it a unique smell and healing qualities. Treating digestive problems is one of the most well-known uses for peppermint oil. Its gastrointestinal tract-soothing effects have led to its use in the treatment of bloating and other symptoms associated with irritable bowel syndrome (IBS).

Due to its analgesic qualities, peppermint oil is often used to treat headaches and migraines. Its uses don't stop with internal consumption; diluted, it can be administered externally to relieve tense and painful muscles.

In addition, the invigorating scent of peppermint oil has been linked to enhanced mental focus and alertness, which is why aromatherapists frequently use it.

TURMERIC AND CURCUMIN

Due to its possible health benefits, turmeric, a vivid yellow spice, has long been used in traditional medicine. Curcumin is the active ingredient that is in charge of many of its medicinal actions. Curcumin, well-known for its strong antioxidant and anti-inflammatory qualities, has been researched for its potential to treat several illnesses, including cardiovascular disease and arthritis.

Turmeric, which is frequently used in cooking, gives food a subtle flavor and bright color. Its medical application goes beyond the kitchen, though. It has demonstrated promise in lowering inflammation, promoting joint health, and maybe delaying cognitive decline. Although curcumin is present in turmeric, its bioavailability is restricted. Therefore, supplements containing curcumin are available to offer this advantageous component in a more concentrated and easily absorbed form.

A trifecta of herbal medicines with a variety of uses in health and wellness are aloe vera, peppermint oil, and turmeric with curcumin. With applications ranging from headache relief to inflammation management, and from skincare to digestive health, these natural remedies are still drawing interest due to their capacity to improve overall health. As with any herbal therapy, it's important to use them sparingly, taking into account specific medical concerns and seeking professional advice as needed.

CHAPTER SEVEN

GUT HEALTH AND PROBIOTICS: AN OVERVIEW OF THE GUT MICROBIOME

The complex collection of bacteria, viruses, fungi, and other microorganisms that live in the gastrointestinal system is referred to as the gut microbiome. This complex ecosystem affects many physiological systems, which is essential for preserving general health. Trillions of bacteria, totaling around 2 kg, are present in the human stomach. These microorganisms support immune system regulation, nutrition absorption, and digestion.

The gut microbiome's composition is very dynamic and impacted by a variety of factors, including lifestyle, environment, genetics, and food. Better health outcomes are connected to a diversified and healthy microbiome, while imbalances in this ecosystem have been linked to several illnesses, such as obesity, autoimmune disorders, and inflammatory bowel diseases.

IBS PROBIOTIC STRAINS

Symptoms of the common gastrointestinal illness known as Irritable Bowel Syndrome (IBS) include bloating, irregular bowel habits, and abdominal pain. Probiotics have drawn attention to their ability to treat IBS symptoms. Probiotics are described as live bacteria that, when given in sufficient concentrations, impart health benefits.

Numerous probiotic strains have been effective in reducing symptoms associated with IBS. Probiotics for IBS that are most researched and commonly utilized include Lactobacillus and Bifidobacterium species. These strains may improve the function of the gut barrier, lower inflammation, and modify the gut microbiota to achieve their desired effects. Clinical trials have demonstrated improvements in bloating, bowel habits, and abdominal pain in IBS patients who took particular probiotic formulations.

It's crucial to remember that different people will respond to probiotics differently, and the strains that work best for you may vary depending on your particular IBS symptoms and underlying causes. Furthermore, research is still being done to determine the best probiotic supplement dosage and duration for managing IBS.

FERMENTATION FOODS

Since ancient times, humans have included fermented foods in their diets, and these items are essential for supporting gut health. Microorganisms such as bacteria, yeast, and molds convert sugars and carbohydrates during the fermentation process. This process of transformation produces useful substances including probiotics, vitamins, and bioactive peptides in addition to extending the shelf life and flavor of food.

Fermented foods include things like yogurt, kefir, sauerkraut, kimchi, and miso. The diversity and equilibrium of the gut microbiome are enhanced by the abundance of living beneficial bacteria found in these foods. Frequent use of fermented foods has been linked to better immune system function, better digestion, and increased nutritional absorption.

Fermented foods frequently contain bioactive substances with anti-inflammatory and antioxidant properties in addition to probiotics. These substances may also improve general health and aid in the treatment or prevention of several gastrointestinal conditions.

Maintaining optimal gut health requires knowing the complexities of the gut microbiome, investigating probiotic strains for managing IBS, and including fermented foods in the diet. These fields are seeing a growth in research that is illuminating the complex interactions between human health and the microbiome.

CHAPTER EIGHT

CHANGES IN LIFESTYLE

STRESS MANAGEMENT

Keeping a healthy lifestyle requires effective stress management. People frequently deal with a variety of stressors in today's fast-paced environment, which can have a detrimental effect on their physical and mental health. To lessen these difficulties, appropriate stress management strategies must be adopted. Strategies like time management, mindfulness, and reaching out to others for support can help people manage their stress and avoid the negative consequences it can have on their health.

MIND-BODY METHODOLOGIES

The focus of mind-body approaches is on the relationship between the mind and body, acknowledging that mental and emotional wellness can have a major influence on physical health.

Mind-body therapies that support relaxation and general well-being include progressive muscle relaxation, guided imagery, and meditation. These methods help to increase mental clarity and emotional resilience in addition to reducing stress.

YOGA AND MEDITATION

Due to their numerous holistic health advantages, these age-old activities have become increasingly popular. Yoga enhances physical strength, flexibility, and mental focus by combining physical postures, breath control, and meditation. In contrast, profound concentration and awareness are key components of meditation, which promotes inner calm and harmony. Including yoga and meditation in your daily practice can improve your general well-being and be a very effective way to reduce stress.

BREATHING TECHNIQUES

In the yogic tradition, conscious breathing techniques, or pranayama, are a key component of stress reduction and relaxation. Deep breathing exercises that trigger the relaxation response in the body, such as diaphragmatic and alternate nostril breathing, can lower stress levels and heart rates. Regularly including breathing exercises in one's regimen can be a straightforward yet powerful way to reduce stress and encourage mental calmness.

PHYSICAL ACTIVITY AND EXERCISE

One of the main components of a healthy lifestyle is regular exercise. There are several advantages to physical activity, such as better weight management, elevated mood, and improved cardiovascular health. Exercise helps reduce stress by fostering a sense of well-being and success, which produces endorphins, the body's natural mood enhancers.

Finding fun ways to exercise is essential to maintaining a long-term commitment to physical activity, whether that means walking, cycling, or playing team sports.

ADVANTAGES OF FREQUENT EXERCISE

Frequent exercise has advantages that go beyond improved physical health. Exercise has been shown to enhance cognitive performance, enhance the quality of sleep, and lessen anxiety and depressive symptoms. It is also essential for preserving a healthy weight and lowering the chance of developing chronic illnesses. Developing a regular exercise regimen is a highly effective means of improving general well-being and cultivating an optimistic outlook.

ACTIVITIES THAT ARE GOOD FOR PEOPLE WITH IBS

When it comes to exercise, people with Irritable Bowel Syndrome (IBS) frequently encounter particular difficulties. Patients with IBS may benefit from low-impact exercises like walking, swimming, and light yoga since they are less likely to cause gastrointestinal distress. People with IBS must pay attention to their bodies and select activities that enhance their well-being without aggravating symptoms. Getting advice from medical professionals can assist in customizing a fitness program to meet the unique requirements of people with IBS.

FORMULATING AN INDIVIDUALIZED WORKOUT PROGRAM

Personalized workout plans are created by taking into account each person's preferences, degree of fitness, and health objectives. Whether the goal is stress management, weight loss, or cardiovascular health enhancement, a personalized program should combine strength, flexibility, and aerobic training. Consistency and gradual advancement are essential components of any successful fitness program. Creating a customized strategy that fits a person's particular lifestyle and health goals can be greatly aided by consulting with fitness experts or healthcare doctors.

CHAPTER NINE

INTEGRATIVE METHODOLOGIES
THE USE OF ACUPUNCTURE

An essential part of integrative healthcare methods that are based on traditional Chinese medicine is acupuncture. This traditional method entails inserting tiny needles into predetermined bodily locations to restore equilibrium to the body's Qi, or energy flow. The foundation of acupuncture theory is the idea of Qi, and numerous health problems are thought to result from disturbances in its flow. Acupuncturists aim to encourage natural healing processes and restore equilibrium in the body by stimulating certain areas.

HOW THE HERB WORKS

Although the workings of Western medicine do not fully understand the mechanism underlying acupuncture's benefits, several ideas try to explain them.

One theory is that endorphins and other neurotransmitters that reduce pain and enhance well-being are released when nerves, muscles, and connective tissues are stimulated. Furthermore, acupuncture may affect the autonomic nerve system, which could affect processes like digestion and blood pressure. Numerous studies indicate that acupuncture can be useful in addressing a range of diseases, including chronic pain, nausea, and musculoskeletal disorders, however, the exact processes underlying its effectiveness are still being investigated.

STUDIES AND PROOF

The effectiveness of acupuncture has been the subject of increasing research and evidence in recent years, which has helped to legitimize it as a therapeutic tool. Its efficacy in treating ailments like osteoarthritis, migraines, and chronic pain has been investigated in numerous clinical trials. Even though the results are frequently contradictory, some research indicates that acupuncture can be a beneficial addition to traditional medical treatments. Moreover, research suggests that acupuncture may have a role in modifying the immune system and lowering inflammation, suggesting potential advantages for illnesses having an inflammatory component.

HOMEOPATHY

Homeopathy is another integrative approach rooted in alternative medicine principles. Founded by Samuel Hahnemann in the late 18th century, homeopathy is based on the concept of "like cures," where substances that cause symptoms in a healthy person are used in highly diluted forms to treat similar symptoms in a sick person. Homeopathic remedies are prepared through a process of potentization, which involves successive dilution and succussion (vigorous shaking).

PRINCIPLES OF HOMEOPATHIC TREATMENT

The principles of homeopathic treatment extend beyond addressing specific symptoms; practitioners consider the individual's overall constitution and the unique way in which symptoms manifest. The goal is to stimulate the body's vital force, allowing it to restore balance and initiate the healing process. While the underlying principles of homeopathy differ significantly from conventional medicine, some individuals find relief from various ailments through homeopathic treatments.

COMMON REMEDIES FOR IBS

In the context of integrative approaches to gastrointestinal health, homeopathy offers potential solutions for conditions like Irritable Bowel Syndrome (IBS). Common homeopathic remedies for IBS include Nux vomica, Lycopodium, and Pulsatilla, among others. These remedies are chosen based on the individual's specific symptoms and constitution. While the scientific basis for homeopathy is a subject of debate, some patients report positive outcomes and ongoing research continues to explore its potential benefits and mechanisms of action.

Integrative approaches often emphasize the importance of individualized care, acknowledging that different modalities may resonate with different individuals based on their unique health profiles and preferences.